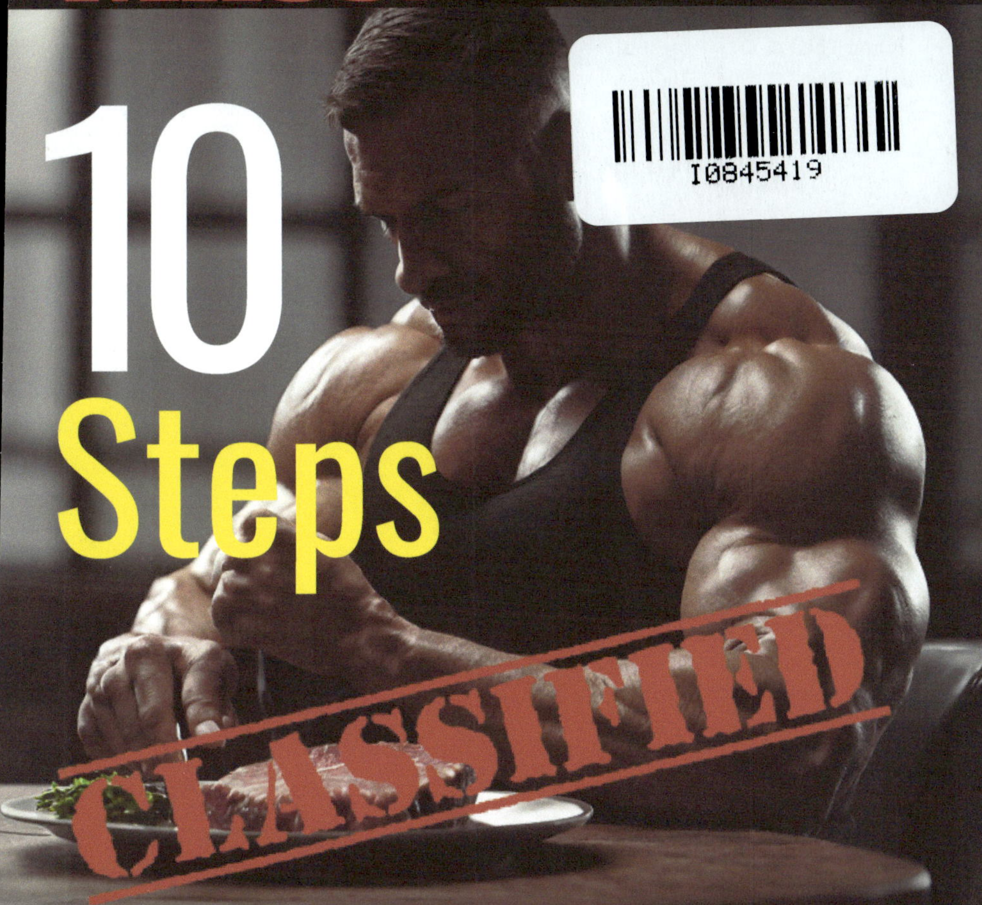

UNLOCKING THE SECRETS TO GAINING MASS!
10
Steps
I0845419
CLASSIFIED
TO ACHIEVING YOUR DREAM SIZE!

# Table of Contents

INTRODUCTION

# Hello, my name is Glory and I'm here to serve.

I've been passionate about weightlifting for as long as I can remember. I believe I was 9 when I got my first 5-pound cast iron dumbbell' set. Man were those things heavy! lol After that I was sold on getting swole. With determination and discipline, I worked out regularly only to learn that my genetics and extremely fast metabolism would betray me, putting me on a 12-year trajectory of struggle and frustration to pack on the pounds. Sound familiar?

I graduated high school standing at 6'1 and a whopping 165 pounds. If I had a penny for every time I was told "you would blow over in a strong wind" or every time someone whistled when I took my shirt off. Not for the reason one might wish for, but to tell me to put that bird back in his chest! Lol I laugh now but back then it was no laughing matter.

In my 30 years of body building, I've discovered the ten most effective steps anyone can implement to achieving their weight gain goals. When I started doing these 10 things, I grew 100% natty! If you start doing these 10 things NOW, the potential to put on size you never had before is great. It will take discipline and commitment on your part.

Some of you may not even be into fitness but just want to put a little meat on the bones.

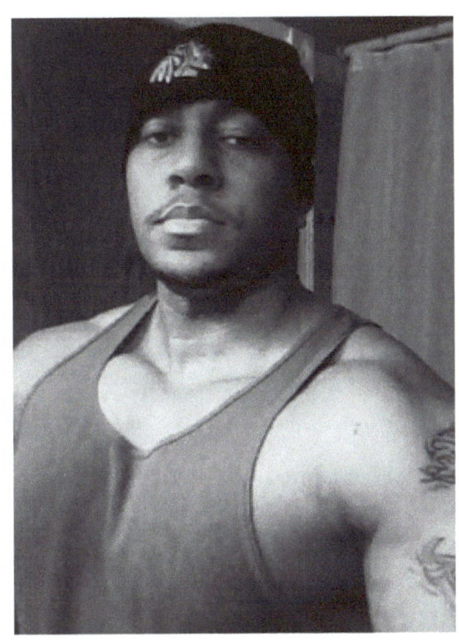

It doesn't matter male or female, bodybuilder, workout warrior or couch potato, if your issue is putting on size, I've got the solution to get you the breakthrough you've been praying for!

# -Glory

CHAPTER I.1

# Mathematics

### Common Misconceptions

Before delving into the specifics of weight gain, it's crucial to dispel common misconceptions:

**Misconception 1:** "Weight gain is solely about getting fat." This is far from the truth. Gaining weight should focus on increasing lean muscle mass, not just adding excess body fat.

**Misconception 2:** "Eating anything will help you gain weight." While calories are essential for weight gain, the quality of those calories matters. A diet consisting of junk food may lead to unhealthy weight gain and negatively impact your health.

### The Science of Weight Gain

Weight gain, fundamentally, comes down to a simple concept: caloric intake versus caloric expenditure. If you consume more calories than your body burns, you will gain weight. To better understand this process, let's explore some key terms:

**Caloric Surplus:** To gain weight, you need to create a caloric surplus, which means consuming more calories than your body needs for its daily functions and activities. This excess energy is used to build and repair tissues, including muscle.

**Pro Tip: Search google for a free TDEE calculator.**

**Basal Metabolic Rate (BMR):** BMR represents the number of calories your body needs to maintain its basic functions at rest, such as breathing, circulation, and cell production. It varies from person to person and is influenced by factors like age, gender, and genetics.

**Total Daily Energy Expenditure (TDEE):** TDEE accounts for all the calories your body burns throughout the day, including those used for physical activity, digestion, and metabolism. It's calculated by adding your BMR to the calories burned through daily activities and exercise.

**Thermic Effect of Food (TEF):** TEF refers to the energy expended during digestion, absorption, and utilization of food. Different macronutrients (proteins, carbohydrates, and fats) have varying TEF values.

**Body Composition:** Gaining weight should primarily involve increasing lean muscle mass rather than body fat. Your body composition is the ratio of muscle to fat, and it's an essential aspect of your fitness journey.

Understanding these concepts will help you make informed decisions about your calorie intake, exercise regimen, and overall strategy for healthy weight gain but for now let's summarize and map out a plan of action.

CHAPTER 1.2

# Mathematics

**Learn To Count**

## Step # 1: Eat at a caloric surplus daily!

2+2 =4 and 3+ 1 equals 4 also. It never equals 5 or any other number. In other words if you take the number of calories your body uses a day and add a surplus of calories in addition to that number, you will gain weight. It's simple math.

Some of you might say " I tried that already and it doesn't work." Here are 2 key reasons why it hasn't.

Reason 1

- **The calculator, chart or process you used to determine your TDEE is wrong.**

In other words, for example you thought your body burns 2000 calories a day so you increased your caloric intake by 300 calories a day. When in reality your body might burn 2300 calories a day so the extra 300 calories or so you thought, are actually just helping you maintain the weight you have.

This means that you would have to consume more than 2300 calories to be at a surplus and effectively gain more weight.

The issue is most TDEE calculators are only estimates. Tools to help put you in the ball park of how many calories you burn per day however, there are many variables that come into play when calculating, that could make these calculators inaccurate.

The more calories you intake in addition to your TDEE the faster you will gain weight. The goal is to **consume 1000 more calories** than you burn on a daily bases. If your body burns 2300 calories in a day then you should consume 3300 calories a day.
This is the optimal solution to put on weight in the quickest time possible. Now if you're gaining faster than you want, you can cut the surplus calories down as you see fit.

You might be thinking how am I going to put down 1000 extra calories on top of the calories I need to sustain?

It's actually easy once you have the knowledge and systems in place. This is why this book exists. You're in good hands!

CHAPTER 1.3

# Mathematics

Reason 2:

- **The calculation of the amount of calories you THINK you're taking in is wrong.**

Again, it's mathematics. Either you aren't counting your calories for all the food you intake for the day or you flunked math like I did lol!

Many times the issue is that we just get lazy and don't feel like continuously counting calories all day so we slack and just assume we might have met our goal.

Unless you are rich, if you are, can I borrow a dollar? You don't have an extensive variety of exotic meal choices from day to day.

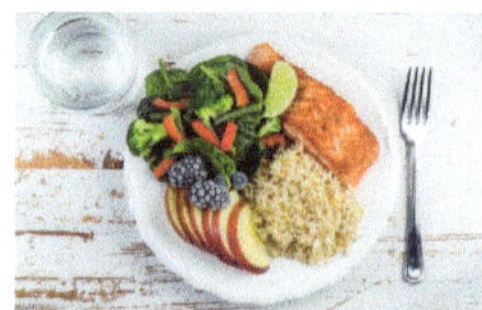

This means that the meals you eat the most are probably only a handful. So do the work now. Think about the meals you will be eating on a regular basis and figure out the calories and proportions you need.

**FATSECRET.COM** is a free website that can help you identify how many calories are in various food products.

When you meal prep, which we will cover later, this will come in handy and once familiar with the calorie count, you will automatically know how many calories for certain dishes and snacks. This will help you to stay on target with your calorie goals without having to count every single meal.

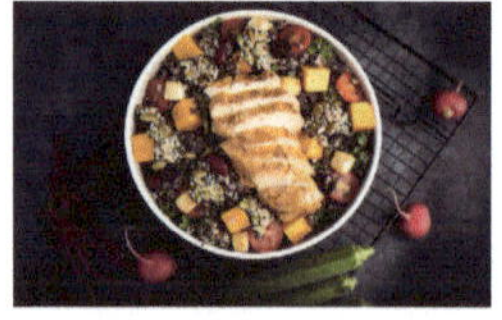

Try planning 4 big meals a day with high calorie snacks in-between. So you will split your calorie goal i.e. 3300 calories a day, into 4 meals including snacks.

Here is an example of a 3300 calorie meal split.

CHAPTER 1.4

# Mathematics

BREAKFAST: 900 CALORIES
SNACK: 200 CALORIES
LUNCH: 800 CALORIES
SNACK 200 CALORIES
DINNER 900 CALORIES
SNACK:300 CALORIES TOTAL = 3300 CALORIES

WHAT FOODS SHOULD I CONSUME?

Great question. **Breakfast** is kind of a wild card. Many different choices. Oatmeal, eggs, turkey sausage, whole grain waffles, fruits, nuts, yogurt etc.

It also depends on your schedule and how much time you have in the morning. My breakfast tends to look like this most days.

HIGH CALORIE PROTIEN/WEIGHT GAINER SHAKE – 1000 CALORIES
2 SLICES OF RASIN BREAD BUTTERED – 250 CALORIES
TOTAL CALORIES = 1250

I'll switch it up from time from time to time however the gem is the high calorie shake that makes it easy for me to have a great start towards caloric surplus for the day.

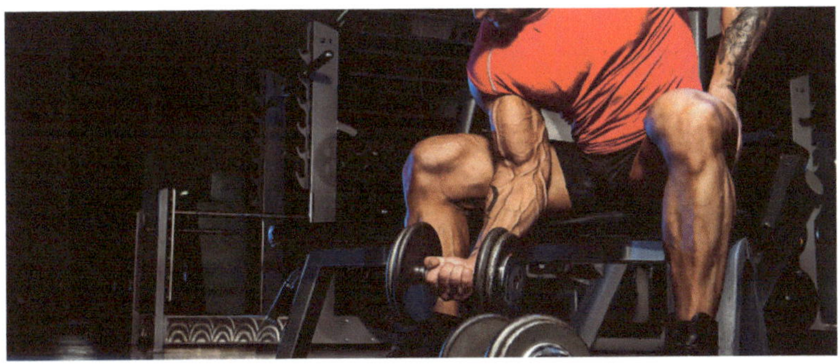

CHAPTER 1.5

# Mathematics

For lunch and dinner I tend to stick with the basics.

**Proteins:**
Chicken
Fish
Turkey
Some red meats. (on occasion)
Beans

**Carbs:**
White/brown rice
Sweet potatoes
Fruits/veggies

These are not including the snacks. There is a special chapter dedicated to that.

## Pro Tip:

Drink whole milk when ever possible. You want to keep your body hydrated by drinking at least a gallon of water a day however for meals, skip the juice and water and go for a nice tall glass of milk. Milk is high in calories as well as a good source of calcium and vitamin D. Unless of course you are drinking a protein shake with your meal which you should always mix your shakes with whole milk, not water for added calories.

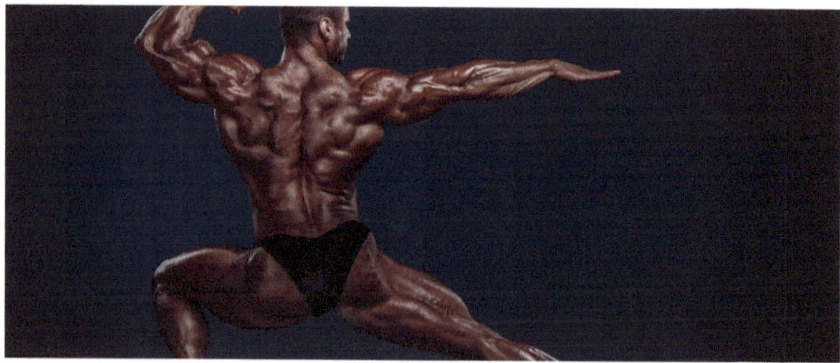

CHAPTER 2:1

# Bird Is The Word

## Step #2: Increase your appetite!

Have you ever heard the term "you eat like a bird?" My mom used to tell me that all the time. What she basically meant was that I didn't have a big appetite so I didn't eat a lot. She was right. The interesting fact that I recently found out, however, is that birds usually eat twice their body weight in a day. So in reality, if I did eat like a bird back then, I would have been massive.

The point is that for many who struggle to put on size, do so because they don't eat enough which is what we covered in the previous chapter, however, many don't eat enough because they just have no appetite.

There are those who eat a ton and still have little to no gain. These are those who have a crazy fast metabolism and their TDEE is much higher than they think it is, therefore not consuming enough calories.

What if I told you I had a top-secret tip that has the potential to double your appetite? Would this book be worth it? I believe so. Let's open the classified document "Project Lettuce."

PROJECT LETTUCE

As I mentioned in my introduction, I've been working out for over 30 years. In that time, I came up with a theory that I knew was true but never really heard talked about amongst the bodybuilding circle I was in.

It wasn't until one late night while watching a random documentary about world record holders that it smacked me in the face. There was a young Oriental man who held the record for winning the most food eating contests.

He was a slender man and was asked by the reporter, how can someone so thin eat that much food? What came out of his mouth was my eureka moment and it solidified my theory after all these years.

"Lettuce!" he said. He then proceeded to tell the reporter that he would take bags and bags of lettuce and roll it up in a certain way and eat them roll by roll and bag by bag. He said the reason he does this is to STRETCH his stomach. The more his stomach stretches, not only the larger capacity to fit food but also because his stomach is used to the volume of food, it expects it, and rumbles when it's not being full to capacity.

CHAPTER 2:2

# Bird Is The Word

He said the reason he does this is to STRETCH his stomach. The more his stomach stretches, not only the larger capacity to fit food but also because his stomach is used to the volume of food, it expects it, and rumbles when it's not being full to capacity.

I never competed professionally so there was no pressure to be consistent or maintain a certain size all the time. So there would be periods where I would slack on the caloric surplus diet and hitting the gym hard.

When ever I would take time off I always noticed it was a struggle to get back to my diet plan when I started back. My appetite had shrunk because my stomach had shrunk. My stomach had shrunk because I stopped putting a high volume of food in it therefore my appetite went back down to what it normally is which isn't that big.

I learned in order to kick start my appetite, I had to stretch my stomach again to the point that it would crave large volumes of substance just to keep from grumbling.

The easiest way I found to stretch my stomach is to drink large high calorie protein shakes. I'm not talking monstrously large like these 32 to 40 oz. shakes that you see some weight lifters drink. I'm talking a 20 to 24 oz. shake.

Drinking 2 of these shakes a day and forcing at least 2 additional 800-900 calorie meals, so 4 meals total, was enough to stretch my stomach back out within 2 weeks.

Yes those two weeks are uncomfortable and you get that super full feeling however toughen up! Your gains are at stake and it will only be uncomfortable for about two weeks.

After the two weeks, give or take some days, your stomach will go from feeling full to expecting that volume daily. Also if you are eating at the same times ever day, your stomach will act as an alarm and start rumbling when it's close to meal time.

When this switch happens it's game on! You will go from ah man it's time to try to get this shake or meal down to man my stomach is rumbling, I'm so hungry let me feed this beast.

This is when eating becomes more enjoyable and less of a chore and more of a need to keep from feeling hungry BUT...don't fumble the rumble! I'll cover this in the next chapter.

Let's summarize for clarification:

**To increase your appetite you must stretch your stomach.**

CHAPTER 2.3

# Bird Is The Word

To stretch your stomach, you must consume enough food/protein shakes for every meal (at least 4 meals a day) to make you feel full to capacity for at least two weeks, excluding snacks.

The amount of food needed to feel full initially will vary from person to person. The goal is to make sure your 4 meals are measured out calorie wise to evenly distribute the goal number of calories you are aiming to consume daily after calculating what your TDEE is and the surplus calories needed to gain weight.

Remember everyone's body composition is different as well as everyone's goals.

A 5'5 female weighing 125 pounds is not going to need to consume 3300 calories a day to gain weight.

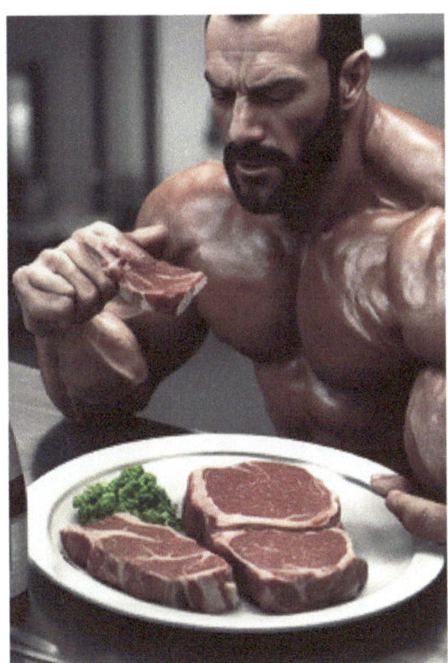

The objective is to be able to consume the meals you have determined you need per day to meet your calorie goal without struggling to do so.

For those who struggle to do so, stretching the stomach will help get you to a place where it's no chore to consume what you need to per meal.

Let-us catch up to these gains! Gain Gains!

Pro Tip: Schedule your meals around the same time ever day and your stomach will let you know when it's time to eat like an alarm clock.

CHAPTER 3

# Fumble Of The Rumble

## Step # 3: When your stomach growls make sure you eat!

As we learned in the previous chapter, stretching our stomachs is a great way to kick-start our appetite. When we successfully do this and eat at regular times every day, our stomachs will rumble like clockwork when it's time to eat.

With this in mind, it's important not to miss the moment when your stomach growls. You may be wondering what this means- it simply means that when your stomach tells you it's empty and ready to eat, you should feed it. Fumbling the rumble happens when you haven't meal planned and have nothing available to eat during this crucial time.

If you fail to plan your meals, you'll most likely end up going hungry until you can get a meal or you'll reach for anything available to eat and snack on. This can lead to bad eating habits and consuming non-quality calories, which can have several negative effects.

The most obvious effect is that eating unhealthy junk food can lead to unwanted fat in unwanted areas. Additionally, it means that you will be behind on your caloric surplus intake and will most likely be scrambling to catch up for the day.

By the way, have you ever wondered why your stomach rumbles?

Here are three major factors:

1.BRAIN SIGNALS OF HUNGER:
THE HYPOTHALAMUS, A PART OF THE BRAIN, DETECTS A DECLINE IN BLOOD GLUCOSE (SUGAR) LEVELS AFTER A PERIOD OF FASTING. THIS IS ONE OF THE PRIMARY CAUSES OF HUNGER.

2. THE "HUNGER HORMONE:
 THE STOMACH LINING RELEASES A HORMONE CALLED GHRELIN IN REACTION TO THE DROP IN BLOOD GLUCOSE LEVELS.  GHRELIN IS FREQUENTLY REFERRED TO BECAUSE IT INCREASES APPETITE AND BLOOD LEVELS BEFORE MEALS. IT WORKS BY SIGNALING THE HYPOTHALAMUS THAT THE BODY NEEDS FOOD.

3. EMPTY STOMACH:
THESE CONTRACTIONS MAY BECOME MORE NOTICEABLE AND AUDIBLE IF THE STOMACH IS EMPTY IN BETWEEN MEALS. THE INTESTINES AND STOMACH KEEP CONTRACTING AS THEY "CLEANSE" THEMSELVES OF ANY LEFTOVER FOOD OR GAS.

IN SUMMARY, DON'T FUMBLE THE RUMBLE!

CHAPTER 4.1

# You Snooze You Lose

## Step #4: Meal Prep Meal Prep Meal Prep!

Now that we understand that "to not fumble the rumble" means to always have quality high-calorie food available, we can talk about how to prepare ourselves to never fumble the rumble again. The key is meal prep.

You've probably heard this before, but how many of us who struggle to put on weight actually meal prep all our meals so that we always have food available? If we're honest with ourselves, not many. But meal prep is a simple concept that is crucial if we want to successfully put on size on a consistent basis.

When I don't meal prep properly, I know I'm going to have a bad week in terms of hitting my caloric surplus goals, or I might end up eating foods I shouldn't. But when I make sure to meal prep at the beginning and middle of the week, I almost always hit my goals, which leads to positive weight gain.

Here's how I meal prep: I start on Sunday, which is both the beginning of the week and the day I do my grocery shopping. Before I go to the store, I make a grocery list, which helps me avoid spending long hours mindlessly wandering the aisles and buying unnecessary things. It also helps me stick to my budget.

I usually shop for one week at a time, but you can adjust to your schedule and finances. The important thing is to plan ahead and always have quality, high-calorie food available.

When it comes to meal prep, small plastic Tupperware containers can be useful, especially if you lead a busy lifestyle. Amazon or similar online stores offer the best deals. However, whether or not you need them depends on your daily routine. If you work a regular 9 to 5 job, having meals prepped in small containers can be very helpful. But, if you work from home, you may not need to use them.

Personally, I cook my meals and store them in large containers. Whenever I need to eat I simply take out the required amount and serve it onto my plate. But, if you're looking for more time-saving options, you can put your meals into individual Tupperware containers and store them in the refrigerator, ready to heat and eat. Ultimately, the choice is yours.

CHAPTER 4.2

# You Snooze You Lose

If you're always on the go, then small containers are a must-have. Remember to plan ahead and incorporate your calorie intake goals into your meal planning and grocery list. You've already calculated the number of calories you need to consume daily, and you know what meals you'll be having and how many calories each meal contains.

When you're cooking and meal prepping, keep this in mind. I usually meal prep on Sundays, cooking enough food to last for three days. On the third day, I meal prep again to last another three days, leaving one day for a cheat day. On cheat days, remember to practice portion control. You can indulge in some of your favorite foods, but don't go overboard, or your efforts will be counterproductive.

Not to sound redundant however I will repeat this until you ingrain this in your psyche. One of the most crucial steps that you can take to ensuring a successful path to weight gain is meal prep.

Always making sure that you have food readily available at arm's reach to not only feed your stomach whenever it Rumbles but also times when you're not hungry or full and you can take in those extra calories because it's easily accessible. This is a game changer. I repeat, **this is a game changer!**

It will require discipline however if you do this religiously you will obtain great results. However, if you snooze on meal prepping you will lose. Pun intended.

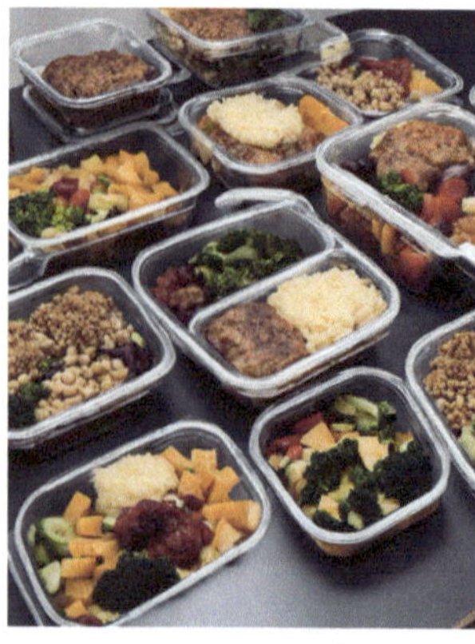

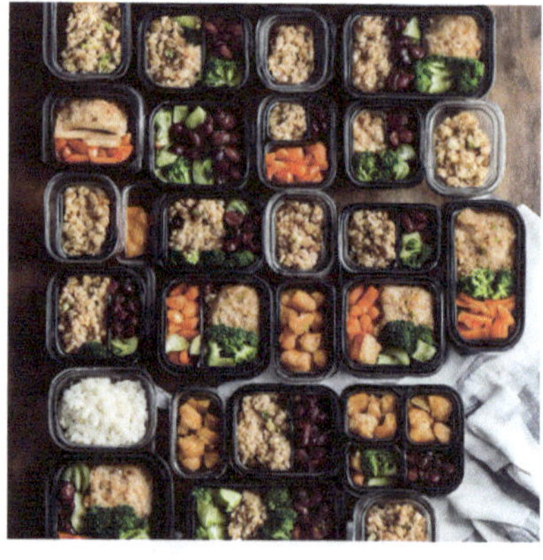

CHAPTER 5

# A Need For Speed

## Step #5: The faster you eat, the more you eat!

So far, we have figured out how many calories we need to gain weight efficiently, how to stretch our stomachs to increase our appetite, and how to take advantage of our appetite by meal prepping.

Here's another top-secret trick that will help you pack in more food, which means packing on more pounds.

Let's take a look at the classified top-secret file "**A Need for Speed**".

When you eat slowly, your body has more time to release hormones that signal fullness, such as leptin. Eating at a moderate pace allows these signals to reach your brain, helping you recognize when you're satisfied, and causing you to stop eating. So, let's reverse-engineer this.

When you eat rapidly, on the other hand, you may consume more calories before your body has a chance to signal to your brain that you're satisfied. The obvious advantage here is that you can put down a larger amount of food before you get that full sensation. This means that you can take in more calories than normal had you ate at a slow or moderate pace.

This is a golden nugget right here, so pay attention and do not take this tip lightly. When implemented, you will drastically see how much more food you're able to consume. You might not win any Best Manners Awards at the dinner table, but boy will you put on weight.

This also goes for protein shakes. One of the main issues I had was downing an ultra-thick 24 oz. protein shake. I would find myself taking between 25 to 30 minutes, sometimes even longer, to finish it. I was sipping it like it was a caramel macchiato from my favorite barista shop.

Once I learned this little trick and was intentional about guzzling the shake immediately after I made it, I would be done in literally 5 minutes or less, which gave me room to add a few extra calories by adding a snack or something else I could munch on if I wanted.

That being said, remember, don't fumble the rumble, so always make sure you have some high-calorie snacks close by. Whether you're drinking your protein shake for a meal, be it breakfast, lunch, or dinner, make sure you have something extra in a Tupperware container in the refrigerator, or some snacks close by, so that you can take advantage of the time window before your hormones tell your brain that you're full.

CHAPTER 6.1

# The Time To Dine

## Step #6 Make sure you eat at the right times!

Any meal counts in the pursuit of gaining mass and muscle, but breakfast is the most important. The foundation of your daily nutrition plan is breakfast, which may make or break your goals. In this chapter, we'll discuss why breakfast matters so much and how it can work wonders.

The Benefit of Breakfast

### 1. Breaking the Fast:

The significance of the term "breakfast" is highlighted. Your body has practically been fasting since your last meal the night before when you get up. Your body receives a signal when you eat breakfast, telling it to transition from a catabolic state—where it breaks down tissue for energy—to an anabolic state—where it builds and repairs tissues. Gaining weight and building muscle require this shift.

### 2. Fueling Your Day:

Breakfast gives you the nourishment and energy you need to start the day off right. It replenishes your glycogen stores, which are necessary for daily activities and exercise. A healthy breakfast keeps you from becoming too tired too quickly and guarantees that you have the energy required for long training sessions.

### 3. Preventing Muscle Catabolism:

As your body looks for nourishment while you sleep, it may go into a moderate condition of protein catabolism. By restoring your levels of amino acids, breakfast helps stop this deterioration of your muscles. This indicates that there are more amino acids available for muscle growth and repair.

### What to include in your Breakfast:

**1. Protein:** The building block of muscle is protein. Muscle growth and recovery are facilitated by eating a healthy breakfast that includes a good supply of protein, such as eggs, Greek yogurt, lean meats, or plant-based alternatives like tofu. Make sure your breakfast contains at least 20–30 grams of protein.

**2. Carbohydrates:** Essential for replenishing your glycogen stores, carbohydrates give you energy. To get consistent energy throughout the day, choose complex carbohydrates like those found in fruits, whole grains, and oats.

CHAPTER 6.2

# The Time To Dine

**3. Healthy Fats:** Nuts, seeds, and avocados are good sources of healthy fats that can help you keep your calorie intake in check and give you sustained energy.

**4. Fiber:** Fiber improves digestion and fullness, which helps you avoid overindulging in harmful snacks later in the day. Increase your consumption of fiber by include whole grains, fruits, and vegetables.

Time Is Important
**1. Pre-Workout Breakfast:** This is very important for people who want to put on weight. Eating a healthy lunch one to two hours prior to working exercise gives you the energy you need to work out effectively. It also prepares the body for post-workout recovery and inhibits muscular catabolism.

**2. Post-Workout Nutrition:** Your muscles are ready for nourishment following a workout. A balance of carbohydrates and protein should be included in your post-workout breakfast to help with muscle regeneration and glycogen replenishment. It's best to have a protein smoothie or a meal that includes balanced carbohydrates and protein.

**Pro Tip:**

**Arrange ahead of time:** Make breakfast the night before to avoid rushing in the morning. This could be a prepared smoothie, overnight oats, or a heated meal. (you snooze you lose!)

The Key is Variety To stay nutrient-rich and avoid boredom, switch up your breakfast selections however don't overwhelm yourself by having to cook 50 different types of meals. Chose a handful you like. Stick with that throughout the month then next month switch it up.

**Remain Hydrated:** Water is vital for healthy digestion and general wellbeing, so remember to drink plenty of it first thing in the morning.

To conclude, breakfast is essential if you want to put on muscle and gain weight. It starts the transition from a catabolic to an anabolic state, giving you the nutrients and energy you require for muscle growth, recuperation, and training. A healthy breakfast lays a solid foundation for the rest of the day and promotes a greater chance of achieving your dream size.

CHAPTER 6.3

# The Time To Dine

Now that we have the most important meal of the day out of the way, let's plan the rest of our meals throughout the day.

You want to make sure that you space out the remainder of your meals evenly. Keep in mind your calorie surplus goal for the day.

By now you should already have a meal plan with all your meals prepped and ready to go. Also, have high-calorie-dense snacks in between meals at hand.

Spread these meals out evenly throughout the rest of the day keeping in mind when you'll have time to eat based on the various tasks and assignments you might have for the day.

Besides breakfast, there are two more crucial times that you want to make sure that you eat. Post-workout as we covered and the last time is right before you go to bed.

Remember as you sleep and your body is in a fasted state you could go into a mild catabolic state. To help combat this it's very important that you eat a heavy meal closer to the time before you get ready to go to bed.

Let's say you eat dinner at 8:00 p.m. however, you don't go to bed until midnight. That's 4 hours past the time you've eaten not to mention the 8 hours of rest you'll be getting. That's potentially 12 hours without refueling your body.

If you go to bed at midnight eat at 11:00 pm. You get the point.

A great way to achieve this is simply by drinking a protein shake right before you go to bed. I usually drink a high-calorie protein shake right before I brush my teeth and then it's off to bed from there. That high-calorie shake sits in my stomach and helps fuel my body while I'm in a fasted sleep.

To summarize, the times that you eat are almost just as important as what you eat and how much you eat. Make sure you're off to a great start and the best chance for success by eating a healthy calorie rich breakfast as soon as you wake. Followed by high-calorie meals and snacks spread evenly throughout the day. Then finish up with a high-calorie meal or high-calorie protein shake right before bed.

I can just feel the gains already. Are you excited? Gain Gains!

CHAPTER 7.1

# Pack The Snacks

## Step #7 Make sure you always have high-calorie/quality snacks at arms reach.

This chapter will be short and sweet. No pun intended however one of my favorite chapters. I know by now you are learning some gems to catapult you on the road to successful weight gain. Here is another.

I have discussed with you in earlier chapters the significance of always having high-quality, high-calorie snacks on hand. You can research the snacks that are best for you on your own. The effective high-calorie snacks that will get the job done. But I'm going to give you two of my favorite snacks that I've been eating for years because I care about you guys and I want you to not struggle like I did for so long. These snacks have successfully helped me to put on and maintain my weight. Did I also mention that they taste really good?

**Snack #1:**

**Chocolate milk and peanuts.**

Peanuts and chocolate milk, indeed! Some of you may even think, "Hey, I eat those already," after reading that. Others may think, "Oh yeah, that makes sense." That being said, some of you may be a little grossed out LOL. While everyone has different tastes, consider this: do you recall the times when your mother made you peanut butter and jelly sandwiches when you were a child or perhaps even as an adult as I do? (I don't live with my mom.) What beverage paired well with a sticky peanut butter sandwich?

Yes, that's right—milk! Peanut butter and milk go well together and are complementary, so there isn't much of a difference in peanuts.

The fact that both of these foods are still reasonably priced despite inflation makes it even better. When I was on the go, it was easy for me to stop at a gas station, which is conveniently located everywhere you go, and specifically get the 2 for a dollar packs of honey-roasted peanuts. Due to inflation, they are now slightly more, but still not by much. I'll then get a 16-ounce jug of vitamin D chocolate milk from the dairy cooler. These two  items cost me under $5.

It gets even better. Let me start by asking any person, big or small, who can't finish a jug of milk and a pack of 2 for a dollar peanuts? It is my belief that those two tiny bags of peanuts and 16 ounces of milk can be finished by anyone with even the smallest appetites.

CHAPTER 7.2

# Pack The Snacks

Guess how many total calories you would have consumed by just eating those peanuts and that milk? 970 calories! Yes! Almost a thousand calories from a snack from the gas station cost you around $4.

You can't beat that with a stick! Here is the breakdown:

**Protein 39 grams**
**Calories 970**
**Carbs 78 grams**
**Sugar 63 grams**

Some of you may be looking at the sugar in the carbs and think that it's too much. If you have this book that means that you have a really hard time putting on weight you probably have a super fast metabolism like I did so these extra carbs and sugars won't hurt you.

Keep in mind most of your diet is going to be clean excluding all sugary drinks like pop and artificial juices. Cutting out all the sugary snack cakes, chips, and ice cream except maybe a cheat day (in moderation).

Although we aren't dirty bulking which is eating all types of high-calorie food good and bad just to get the calories, we are allowing some extra carbs and some sugars into our diet selectively.

So when I talk about having high-calorie snacks in between meals this is one of the Staples that I go to. As you see you can add virtually a thousand calories with a simple snack that tastes delicious.

**Snack #2:**

**Peanut butter and honey sandwiches.**

By now you're probably guessing I love peanut butter. In actuality, I'm a bit tired of it because I've been eating it my entire life and if I had a penny for every pack of honey-roasted peanuts I've eaten I would be a millionaire by now. That being said it is enjoyable, inexpensive, high protein, and calorie-dense.

I use honey because it's healthier for me and I love the way it tastes. What do I wash down my peanut butter and honey sandwiches with? You guessed it milk! Now if I'm having a peanut butter and honey sandwich for a snack I usually make two sandwiches and drink one 16 oz glass of milk or jug of milk.

CHAPTER 7.3

# Pack The Snacks

Peanut butter and honey sandwiches are also easy to prep and throw in a cooler or a bag wherever you go so you can grab them when it's time for a snack.

My peanut butter and honey sandwiches probably don't look like yours. To get the maximum amount of calories I put two tablespoons of peanut butter on each slice of bread. So if I'm making two sandwiches that's two tablespoons of peanut butter on each slice of bread which means that's eight tablespoons of peanut butter.

I use 100% whole-grain wheat bread. It's healthier for you and I just love the taste. Drizzle a little honey on both sandwiches with a tall glass of milk. Delish!

So let's do the math on two peanut butter sandwiches (2 tbsp. of PB on 4 slices of bread) and a 16 oz. glass of chocolate milk. That's 1450 calories for a snack! This could be a meal replacement or used as an in-between snack.

You see why I like peanuts so much? Here's the breakdown:

**Protein 61 grams**
**Sugar 57 grams**
**Carbs 76**
**Calories 1450**

This is by no means is an exhaustive list of high-calorie snacks however it is what I have found to be one of the most inexpensive calorie-dense easily accessible and quick snacks I have used for many years to help gain and keep my size. Feel free to explore different nuts and yogurts and everything else out there to try.

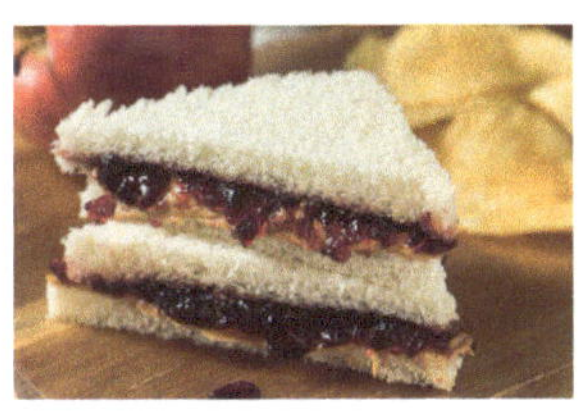

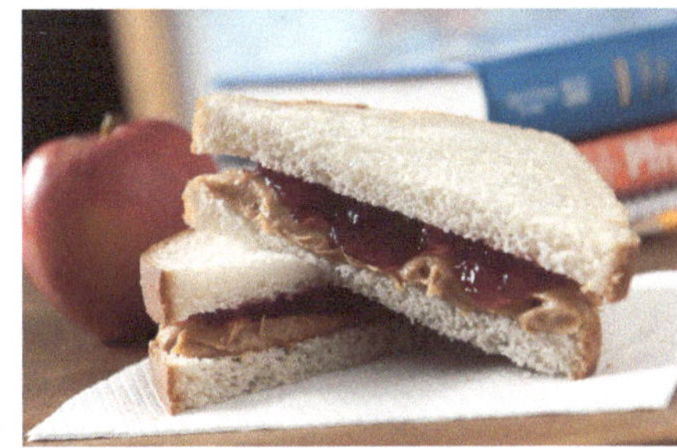

CHAPTER 8.1

# Power In The Powder

## Step #8: It is crucial to take these 2 most important supplements.

To supplement or not to supplement that is the question. Supplement of course! Duh!

This chapter is all about supplements and when I say all about supplements I don't mean an exhaustive list of the 100, supplements that on the market that do various different things. I'm talking about what I use personally and what I have personal experience with.

Everything that I've told you so far has been my personal experience over 30 years of working out. I believe Integrity is law and I would never push or promote something that I haven't taken myself and something that doesn't work.

Full transparency I have no affiliate programs so far with any supplement company. I am not at all opposed to it especially if it's a supplement that I use in that works however I'm simply saying at the time of me writing this there are no agreements but any supplement companies. So what I recommend is solely based off what I use.

There are two supplements that I use that are a must-have for me.

**1. Creatine**

**2. Whey protein**

As I stated in my intro I graduated high school very frail and that was years of me working out trying to put on some Mass. Yes I was ripped but what skinny kid isn't ripped unless you have that body type where you're skinny and hold fat.

After I graduated high school I started to get more serious and more consistent with working out on a regular basis. Went from working out at home with the Raggedy bench in the dumbbells that I've had forever to getting a gym membership and working out in the gym 5 days a week.

With a new wind of motivation and fresh dedication I started to see a little more results but when I say little I mean little!

It wasn't until getting into reading muscle magazines that I came across to supplement called creatine and decided to give it a try. This was a game changer for me.

CHAPTER 8.2

# Power In The Powder

You have to understand that the blueprint that I'm giving you for gaining mass didn't come until years later with trial and error. So the first thing that actually gave me noticeable I should even say drastic results and putting on size and muscle was when I started taking creatine.

Most of you probably already know about creatine many of you might even be on Creatine right now but it is a supplement that if you haven't started yet you need to start. If you are on it, stay on it!

This is one of the supplements clinically tested and proven time After Time to deliver consistent positive results. Of course, I'm referring to Legal supplements.

Make sure you get a jar of creatine monohydrate from a reputable company. The company I use is AllMAX. I've used other brands and haven't had any real issues with them however this is the one that I've stuck with and had great results with.

When I first started using creatine they had many different products that had creatine with a lot of other stuff added a lot of extra sugars added to boost your insulin levels which helps the creatine to absorb in your system. I've learned through experience that you don't need to get the creatine with all the extra bells and whistles. Just get straight creatine monohydrate and drink it with either water or juice. Preferably juice.

Let's get into the gritty little details of creatine.

**Creatine:**

**1. Natural Compound:**

Creatine is a substance that occurs naturally and can be found in small amounts in a variety of foods, with fish, pork, and red meat having the highest concentrations. It is mostly stored in the skeletal muscle of the body, where it is essential for energy metabolism.

**2. ATP and Energy Production:**

The body uses adenosine triphosphate (ATP) as its main source of energy. Adenosine diphosphate (ADP) is a byproduct of the breakdown of ATP during physical activity. ATP is needed for energy production. The body needs to combine ADP with a phosphate group in order to regenerate ATP for ongoing energy supply. Here's where creatine becomes useful.

CHAPTER 8.3

# Power In The Powder

### 3. Creatine Phosphate Reservoir:

Muscle cells store approximately 95% of the body's creatine as creatine phosphate. For brief bursts of high-intensity exercise, like weightlifting, sprinting, or explosive movements, this creatine phosphate reservoir acts as a quick and easy source of phosphate groups to aid in the conversion of ADP back into ATP.

### 4. Enhanced Energy Availability:

Adding creatine monohydrate to a supplement raises the muscle cells' overall creatine phosphate pool. Because of this, ADP can be recycled into ATP more effectively, increasing the body's ability to perform brief bursts of intense exercise. Because of this, people who take creatine supplements frequently report performing better in tasks requiring rapid, intense effort.

### 5. Cell Hydration:

Supplementing with creatine may raise the water content of muscle cells. Improved cell function and muscle growth might be attributed to this cellular hydration. A common side effect of beginning creatine supplementation is a brief increase in body weight due to the increased water content in muscle cells.

### 6. Muscle Growth and Recovery:

Creatine can help with muscle growth and recovery because it improves energy production and cell hydration. In addition to stimulating muscle protein synthesis and enabling you to recover from workouts more quickly, creatine also promotes muscle hypertrophy (growth).

### 7. Dosage and Loading:

The standard dosage for creatine monohydrate entails a "loading phase" during which users take about 20 grams per day (split into 4 doses) for 5-7 days and a "maintenance phase" during which time 3–5 grams per day are adequate. The purpose of the loading phase is to rapidly overload the muscles with creatine, and the maintenance phase keeps those levels stable.

**Pro Tip: Drink your creatine with juice like orange juice or grape juice. The carbs in the juice spike your insulin which helps to absorb creatine into your muscles.**

CHAPTER 8.4

# Power In The Powder

Now that we've covered creatine let's take a look at the second must-have supplement, protein.

I'm sure you've heard this before, protein is the main building block of muscle right? What if I told you that was wrong? If you do a quick Google search they are quick to tell you that muscle is 80% protein however what you fail to realize is how they word it.

They would say phrases like outside of water or other than water muscles are 80% protein. So then how much water is in our muscles?

Are muscles are 76% water! Water is the major component of muscle. This is why I covered creatine first. The volumizing effect of creatine with the ability to hydrate your muscles is the reason why It works so well. This is why it is imperative that you drink at least a gallon of water a day.

If you working out hard and have disciplined yourself with eating at a caloric Surplus yet you're not drinking enough water, you are working against yourself.

When we talk about drinking water for hydration it's not only quenching your thirst but it's also hydrating in the volumizing your muscles. Sprinkle in some magic creatine and protein and poof big beefy muscles!

Now that we have an understanding of how important water is and how water and creatine work hand in hand, let's discuss the second most important building block of muscle, whey protein.

**1. Complete Protein Profile:**

Whey protein has all of the essential amino acids that the body needs, making it a complete protein source. These necessary amino acids are crucial for the synthesis of muscle proteins, which is how new muscle tissue is created. Consuming enough of these amino acids is necessary to promote and sustain the growth of muscle.

**2. Digestion:**

Whey protein is quickly digested and absorbed by the body, making it an excellent choice for post-workout nutrition. Muscles are more sensitive to nutrients after an intense exercise session. Whey protein helps muscles grow and repair during this crucial recovery window by providing a quick supply of amino acids to muscle cells after exercise.

CHAPTER 8.5

# Power In The Powder

Why do I choose whey protein over all the other options? Again I am only going on my PERSONAL experience.

It's what I started using, and what I stuck to. According to the research of professionals, it is the best option for building muscle based on the above facts. It may vary for you.

Soy protein when consumed in large amounts can produce a spike in estrogen production. This is something we want to avoid when trying to pack on the muscle.

To summarize, there are many supplements out there which have many great effects but the two essential supplements which are a must are creatine and whey protein. Using both of these together as directed along with following this 10-step guide to put on size, you are well on your way to achieving the goals that you've been striving so hard to reach.

**Pro Tip: You should be consuming one gram of protein per pound of body weight. So if you weigh 200 lb. you should be taking in 200 g of protein every day. Keep in mind this doesn't have to all come from whey protein shakes. You have to take into consideration that you also get protein from the foods that you eat.**

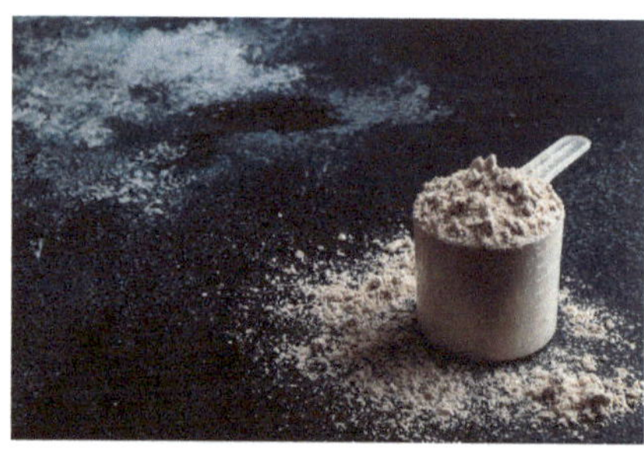

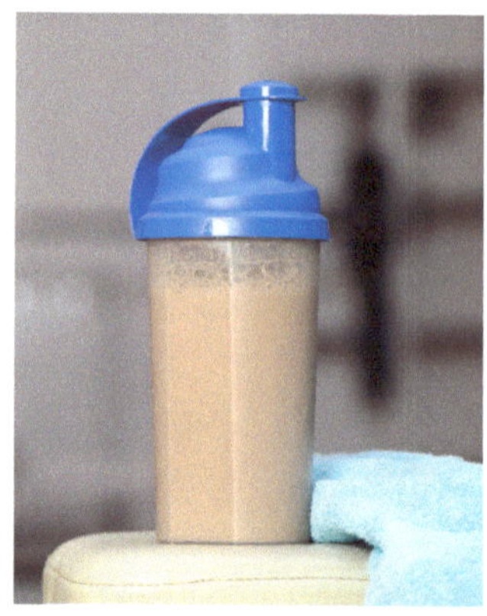

CHAPTER 9.1

# Don't Think It Drink It

## Step #9: Drink half your calories

After studying and watching bodybuilders for many years, I've come to realize that no one is the same however many have some of the same similarities in their process of building muscle and gaining weight.

I'll continue to say this, real food is always better than supplements however many of us including many famous bodybuilders find it easier to meet our caloric goals by drinking a large amount of our calories.

You always want to make sure you're eating enough real foods however if you're like me it's much easier and convenient for me to drink at least half of my calories.

My personal diet plan consists of two 900 to 1,000-calorie meals and two 900 to 1,000-calorie protein shakes with high-calorie snacks in between.

This means I drink almost half of my calories. It's much easier and more convenient for me to do this. It also means less meal prepping which means less cooking and less money spent at the grocery store while still reaching my caloric intake goals.

When it comes to making high-calorie protein shakes there are two ways I go about it.

The first way is to buy a weight-gainer protein product from my favorite supplement company. This option has the whey protein and the calories all packed into one powder. All I have to do is add 16 oz. of vitamin D whole milk for an added 300 calories.

The protein Weight Gainer I've been using for years is by a company called **Universal** in a product called **Real Gains.** As of this moment right now I believe it is being discontinued so I after many years have to search and find an equivalent supplement.

I'm going to reach out to Universal and find out if it's still available. They've been slowly phasing it out. It used to be in supplement stores. Went from supplement stores to only being available online and now the stores that I've been purchasing it from online are saying that it's discontinued.

The reason why I like this protein / Weight Gainer so much is that it wasn't full of unnecessary sugars. It was a clean product. Proper size was not ridiculously big as we see in other protein weight gainers and it only required three and a half scoops for serving size.

CHAPTER 9.2

# Don't Think It Drink It

That three-and-a-half Scoop gives you roughly around 600 calories from the powder alone. Add that to 16 oz. of whole milk a few tablespoons of peanut butter, and whatever fruit you might want to throw in there and you have a thousand-plus calorie shake.

The second way I go about consuming a high-calorie protein shake is I make it myself. That is instead of buying a protein/weight gainer I simply Buy whey protein and then I add the calories to reach my caloric goal of at least 900 to 1000 calories.

Here are the 5 ingredients I use to make this high-calorie shake.

Whey protein (1 serving size)
Peanut butter (2tbsp)
Oats (1/2 cup grounded)
Milk (16 oz.)
Frozen fruit of choice (handful)

Let's start with the Whey Protein. Make sure you get a good quality whey protein from a reputable brand. All whey proteins are not created equal. The amount of protein per serving and the serving size which is usually in scoops, will vary depending on which protein you're using.

I add 16 oz of whole vitamin D milk to a blender or a shaker whichever you prefer. Add the correct amount of scoops of protein for the serving size indicated on the label.

Make sure you get a protein that has a minimum of 30 g of protein per serving. The more grams of protein per serving the better. You don't want to go overboard with the protein however because your body can only process so much protein before it releases the rest as waste.

It's always good to get a protein that has slow and fast-releasing capabilities. This way when you have a shake post-workout you get that immediate protein into the system that's so crucial during the window of time you have and you also get that slower-release protein that continues to feed your muscles over time until your next meal. Always keep that in mind when shopping for a protein or protein / Weight Gainer.

Next add a half cup of oats, 2 tablespoons of peanut butter, and a handful of your favorite Frozen fruit i.e. strawberries or blueberries.

Blend to your liking and enjoy!

CHAPTER 9.3

# Don't Think It Drink It

**Pro tip:** Grind up a large amount of Oats in a high-powered blender and store in an airtight container or gallon Ziploc bag for ease of use when making protein shakes. Grinding oats does not make it lose its nutritional value. It makes for a smoother protein shake with a less gritty consistency. Unless you're someone who likes pulp. In that case no need to grind. Add the oats straight from the canister as they are.

To summarize, if you're having a difficult time prepping all the food required and finding time to sit down and eat four meals a day, it maybe advantageous for you to replace half of your calories with high calorie protein shakes.

Don't think it! Just drink it!

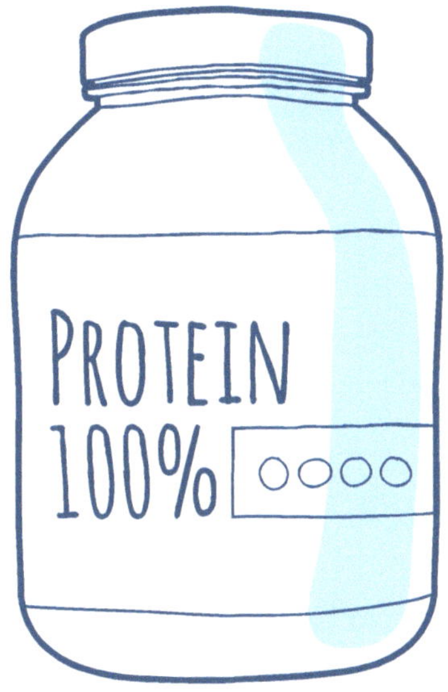


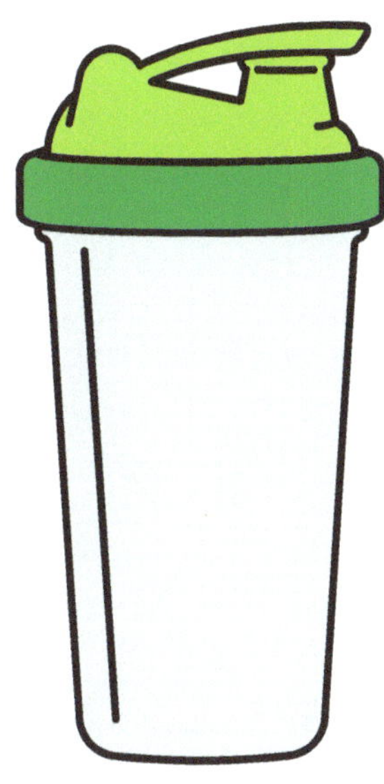

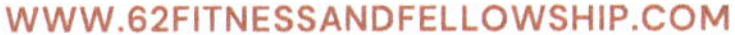

CHAPTER 10

# Med day! Med day!

## Step #10: Consult your physician to make sure there are no medical issues

Med-day Med-day is a play on mayday mayday which is a distress signal.

In this last chapter, I really won't spend a lot of time on them because I hate talking about grim and bad news. After all my goal is to motivate you in a positive way to achieve your dream size that you've been working so hard and so long to achieve.

I'm no Debbie Downer and I never want to rain on anyone's parade so I'll keep this short but not necessarily sweet.

First, let me start by saying that this most likely won't apply to most of you. I believe if you take the 10 steps outlined in this book, you will achieve a high rate of being successful in finally putting on size. However, I have to do my due diligence in discussing a few possible medical reasons that might be keeping you from gaining weight if all else fails.

1. **Hyperthyroidism**

A condition known as hyperthyroidism occurs when the thyroid gland overproduces thyroid hormones, which raises metabolism.
Even with increased calorie intake, this elevated metabolic rate can lead to inadvertent weight loss and make weight gain difficult.

2. **Malabsorption Conditions:**

Several illnesses, including Crohn's disease, IBS, and celiac disease, can make it more difficult for the body to absorb nutrients from food.
Nutrient shortages brought on by malabsorption can cause weight loss or make it difficult to gain weight.

3. **Chronic Illnesses:**

Chronic illnesses such as cancer, HIV/AIDS, and chronic obstructive pulmonary disease (COPD) can cause changes in metabolism, appetite loss, and muscle atrophy, all of which can result in weight loss.

4. **Digestive System Disorders:**

Feelings of fullness can result from conditions like gastroparesis, which causes the stomach to not empty properly, making it difficult to consume enough calories.
Calorie intake and nutrient absorption can also be impacted by chronic diarrhea and inflammatory bowel disease (IBD).

# Conclusion

Are we at the end already? You made it!

I would like to give a big round of applause and congratulate you for investing in yourself and completing this book. I have poured my heart out on these pages and have given you all the information that I know from my personal experience in over 30 years of working out. I know this will get the job done.

Nothing worthwhile comes easy however I am fully persuaded that if you apply these 10 steps with consistency, discipline, and determination, you will achieve amazing results. I can see those gains coming now.

To achieve optimum results, it is assumed that this guide will be accompanied by a healthy resistance training program aka hit the weights! You should be working out at least 3 days a week and a minimum of 45 minutes per workout session.

This gym regimen goes hand in hand with this book and is essential to get optimum results. Subscribe to our website www.62fitnessandfellowship.com for future workout tips and programs to help you get the best out of your workouts.

I would like to take this time to share my heart with you.

Every one of us is fearfully and wonderfully made by God the Father. The world and even ourselves might judge by the outer appearance however God looks at what's in the inside of a person. For it is what is on the inside of a person that is more valuable than outer appearances.

There is nothing wrong with improving our physical temples however we shouldn't let that outweigh our desire to improve what's on the inside. Growing in faith and relationship with God is what's called eternal value.

This comes with the help of God and his holy spirit.

**1 Timothy 4:8**

8 For physical training is of some value, but godliness has value for all things, holding promise for both the present life and the life to come.

I pray you achieve the very best in life and get everything good God has for you. God bless!

**–Glory**

www.ingramcontent.com/pod-product-compliance
Lightning Source LLC
Chambersburg PA
CBHW040318240726
48664CB00006B/1537